KETO CUPCAKE

Discover 30 Easy to Follow Ketogenic Cookbook CupCake recipes for Your Low-Carb Diet with Gluten-Free and wheat to Maximize your weight loss

STEPHANIE BAKER

Copyright © Stephanie Baker

All rights reserved. No part of this book may be reproduced, scanned or distributed in any printed or electronic form without permission. Please do not participate in or encourage piracy of copyrighted materials in violation of the author's rights. Purchase only authorized editions.

1
COCONUT FLOUR AND BLUEBERRY MUFFINS

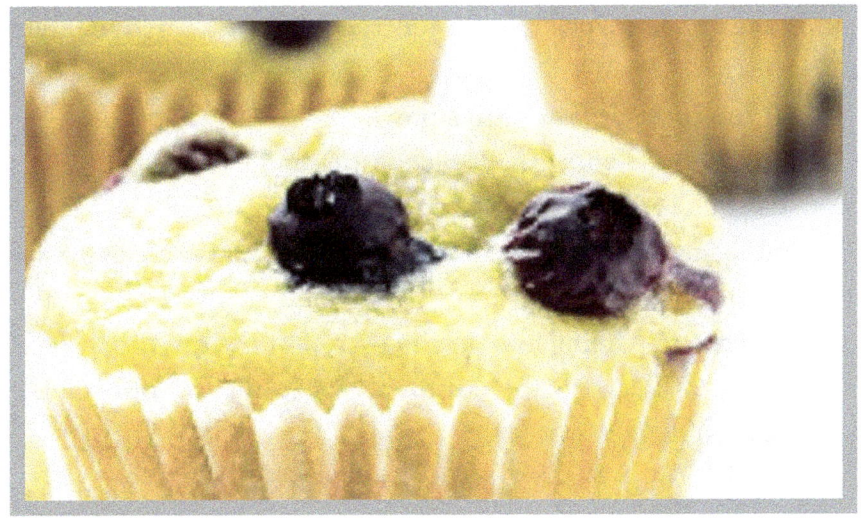

35 MINUTES
Servings 8

. . .

INGREDIENTS

3/4 cup / 75g coconut flour
6 eggs
1/2 cup / 100 g coconut oil, melted
80ml unsweetened coconut or almond milk
1/2 cup / 75g of fresh blueberries
1/3 cup / 40 g granulated sweetener (as fed) or more, to taste
1 teaspoon of vanilla extract or vanilla powder
1 teaspoon of baking powder

PREPARATION

Preheat the oven to 180 degrees Celsius / 356 degrees Fahrenheit.

Sift the coconut flour into a bowl.

Add all ingredients except blueberries and mix well.

Add the blueberries and save some for garnish.

Line a muffin mold with paper cups and fill each cup with batter halfway.

Place the remaining blueberries on top of the muffins.

Bake at 180 degrees Celsius for about 25 minutes or until the surface is golden brown.

DEGREES

For an even lighter batter, you can separate the eggs and beat the egg whites until stiff peaks form. Incorporate the egg whites after mixing the batter. Then add the blueberries last.

If you tend to detect an egg flavor in low-carb baked goods, you can omit 2-3 egg yolks.

You can use frozen blueberries, but fresh ones will blend better and become less mushy.

NUTRITION

Calories: 216 kcal

Total carbohydrates: 7.7 g

Protein: 7.1 g

Fat: 17.1 g

Fiber: 4.3 g

Sugar: 1.7 g

2
STRAWBERRY MUFFIN KETO

KETO CUPCAKE

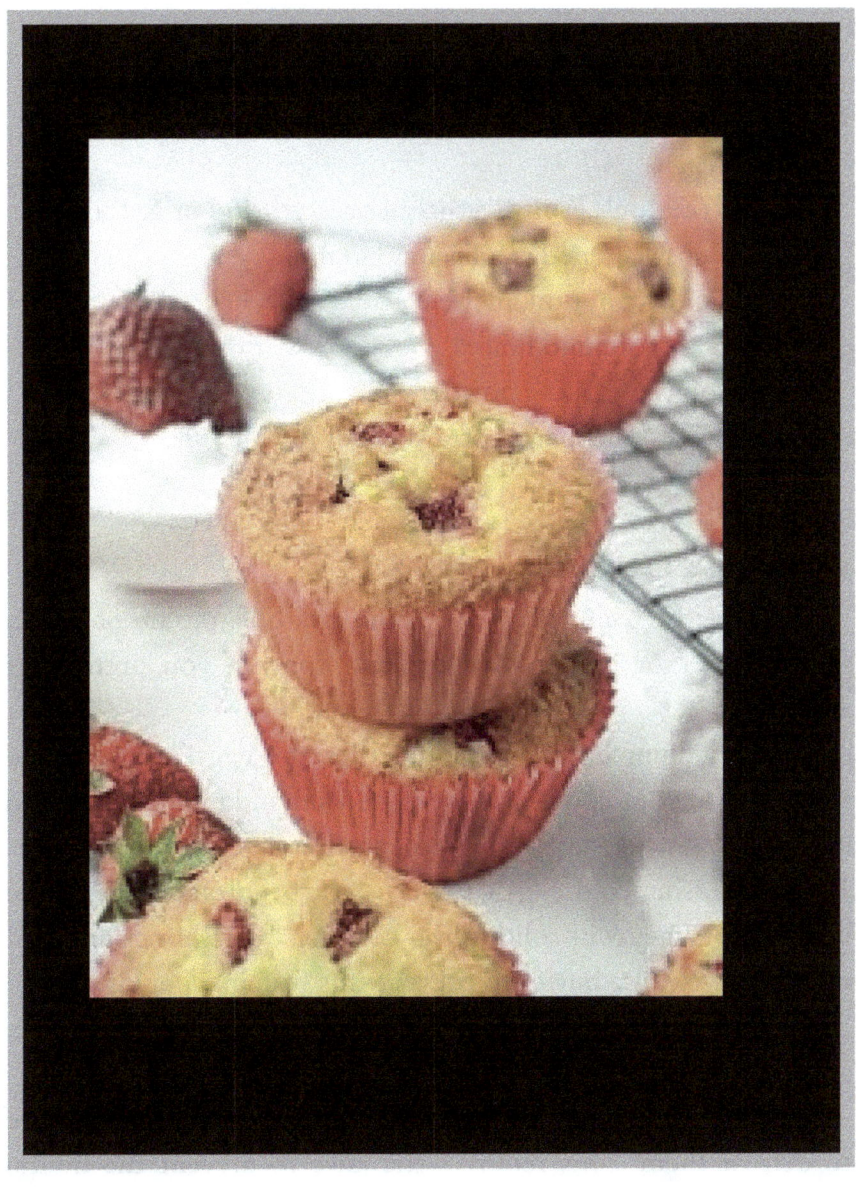

30 MINUTES

Servings 4

INGREDIENTS

- 3 large eggs
- 1/2 cup of Monk Fruit Erythritol or Erythritol or Xylitol
- 1/3 cup unsweetened vanilla almond milk
- 1/3 cup of coconut oil, melted
- 2 1/2 cups of almond flour
- 2 teaspoons of baking powder
- 1 cup of fresh or thawed strawberries (6 ounces)

PREPARATION

Preheat the oven to 180 ° C. Line a 12-hole muffin pan with muffin paper or grease with cooking spray if you prefer. Set aside.

In a medium bowl, whisk together the eggs, unsweetened sweetener of your choice, unsweetened almond milk, and melted coconut oil. Make sure all ingredients are at room temperature. If you are using cold eggs that have just been taken out of the refrigerator, they will solidify the coconut oil creating lumps of oil. Otherwise, use butter to prevent this from happening.

Add the baking powder and almond flour, 1/2 cup at a time, stirring to gently incorporate the flour to avoid lumps.

Add the diced strawberry, if using frozen strawberries be sure to defrost them. This removes the juice to prevent the muffin batter from getting too wet.

Evenly transfer the muffin batter to a 12-muffin tin. I used a mechanical ice cream scoop to be precise and make sure each muffin is the same size (and therefore the same amount of carbs per serving).

Bake for 22-25 minutes or until a toothpick inserted in the center of the muffins comes out clean or with little or no crumbs.

Allow to cool for 10 minutes in the muffin pan, then gently transfer to a wire rack and chill for 30 minutes to 1 hour before eating. Be patient. They get the best consistency at room temperature.

STORAGE

Store in an airtight muffin box for up to 4 days at room temperature.

It can be frozen in airtight zip lock bags, preferably without the paper cup. Defrost the day before at room temperature. It can be toasted or heated in the oven to 100 °C / 210 °F.

HOW TO SERVE YOUR MUFFINS?

Eat on its own or on top with unsweetened coconut whipped cream (or heavy cream) or unsweetened coconut yogurt.

Instruments

3
GLUTEN FREE BLUEBERRY ORANGE MUFFINS

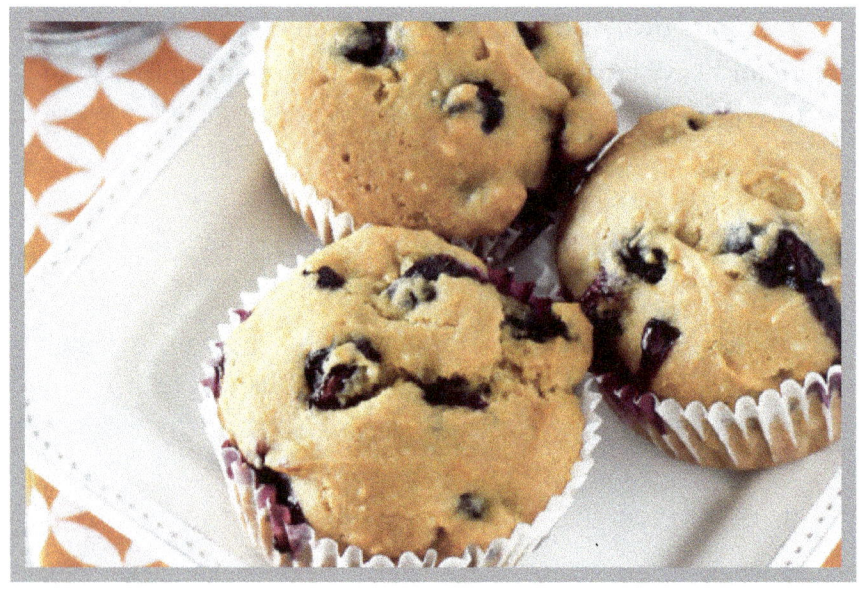

30 MINUTES
servings 6

. . .

INGREDIENTS

For Keto Blueberry Orange Muffins

64 g of almond flour

21 g coconut flour

1 tablespoon psyllium husk

1/2 teaspoon xanthan gum or 2 teaspoons ground flaxseed

1/2 teaspoon baking powder

1/2 teaspoon baking powder

1/4 teaspoon kosher salt

2 egg yolks and the white divided

6 tablespoons to avoid *

2 teaspoons orange zest or 1/4-1/2 teaspoons orange extract

1 teaspoon vanilla extract

1 teaspoon apple cider vinegar

57g organic herb butter melted and slightly cooled

2 tablespoons freshly squeezed orange juice or water

2 tablespoons of water

50-100 g of fresh blueberries to taste (we take as many as possible!)

For the orange glaze

Avoid 3 tablespoons of pastries

1 teaspoon of water

1/2 teaspoon orange zest or orange extract to taste

PREPARATION

Preheat the oven to 180 degrees Celsius. Grease and flour a muffin tin (with coconut flour).

Set aside the egg whites after beating them until soft peaks emerge.

Combine the almond flour, coconut flour, psyllium husk,

xanthan gum, baking soda, baking powder, and salt in a medium mixing bowl. Remove from the equation.

In a large bowl with an electric mixer on medium speed, beat the egg yolks with the sweetener for 1-3 minutes until pale and fluffy.

Add the orange peel (or extract), vanilla extract, vinegar, and melted butter. Slowly add the flour mixture, alternating with water (or orange juice) and whisking until everything is well incorporated.

Gradually add the egg whites to the dough carefully. The batter will be thick at first, but it will melt when you start to beat the egg whites. Add the blueberries.

Spoon batter into prepared muffin pan.

Cook for 18-20 minutes (cover with foil for 13-15 minutes), until golden brown and a toothpick inserted is clean.

ALLOW IT cool in the pan for 15 minutes before taking them out and place them completely in the fridge on a wire rack (they are very tender when hot, so handle them carefully). They will also easily collapse if the blueberries weigh on them.

While the blueberry muffins are cooling, make the orange frosting by mixing the sweetener powder with the orange peel (or extract) and water (or orange juice if desired).

you can Keep for up to 3 days in an airtight bag, but we're fairly sure they'll be gone by then.

OBSERVATIONS

* Or 3 tablespoons of piure. For more information and possible substitutions, see the section on sweeteners.

Please note that the following nutritional information applies to Ketogenic Cranberry Orange Muffins and 2 Tbsp of freshly squeezed orange juice.

4
MONKEY BREAD MUFFIN PUMPKIN SPICE KETO

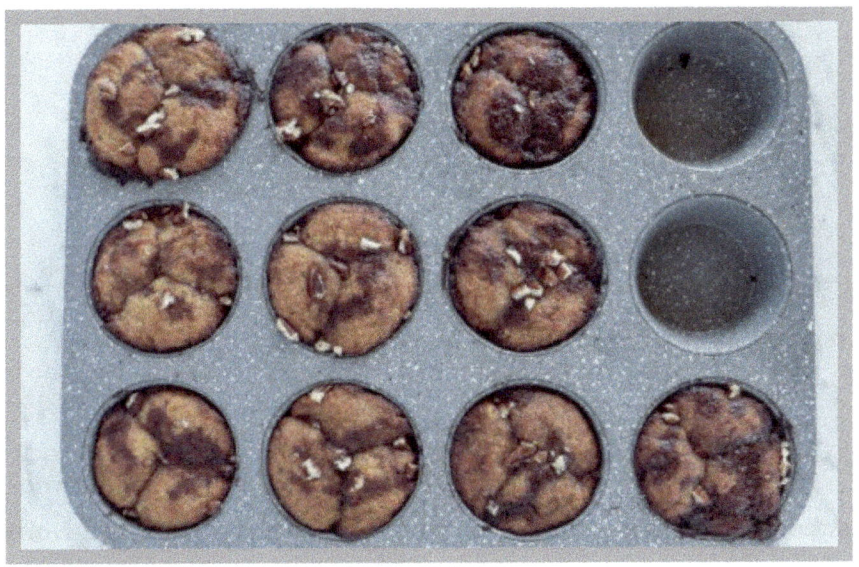

43 MINUTES

Servings 10 muffins

. . .

INGREDIENTS

For pasta:

2 cups whole milk mozzarella, crushed

2 butter spoons

3/4 cup super fine bleached almond flour

1/4 cup coconut flour

2 teaspoons baking powder

3 tablespoons granulated erythritol sweetener

1 teaspoon ground cinnamon

1/8 teaspoon ground nutmeg

1/4 teaspoon allspice

1/4 cup pumpkin puree

2 large eggs

To assemble:

Dodge 1/2 cup

2 teaspoons cinnamon

pinch of salt

2 butter spoons

2 tablespoons chopped pecans (optional)

PREPARATION

For pasta:

Preheat the oven to 350 degrees.

Combine the almond flour, coconut flour, baking powder, sweetener, cinnamon, and nutmeg in a medium bowl and mix well.

Combine the cheese and 2 tablespoons of the butter in a large bowl. Microwave for 2 minutes. Stir well to combine.

Add the dry ingredients, eggs, and pumpkin puree to the melted cheese.

Mix well with a rubber spatula to form a dough. Let the dough rest for 5 minutes.

Meanwhile, grease a muffin tin with butter.

To assemble:

Combine the sweetener, cinnamon, and a pinch of salt in a small bowl and mix well.

Pinch a small piece of dough and roll it into a ball about 4 cm in diameter.

Roll the ball in the sweetener mixture and place in a greased muffin bowl.

Repeat with two more scoops for a total of three scoops per muffin bowl.

Fill the ten cups with three coated dumplings each.

Add the butter to the remaining cinnamon and sweetener mixture and microwave for 30 seconds.

Stir and pour a little of the butter mixture over each muffin.

some chopped walnuts.

Bake in the center of the oven for 30-35 minutes or until golden brown and slightly firm to the touch.

Remove before serving hot and allow to cool slightly.

5

LOW CARB CINNAMON MUFFINS (KETO, PALEO, VEGAN)

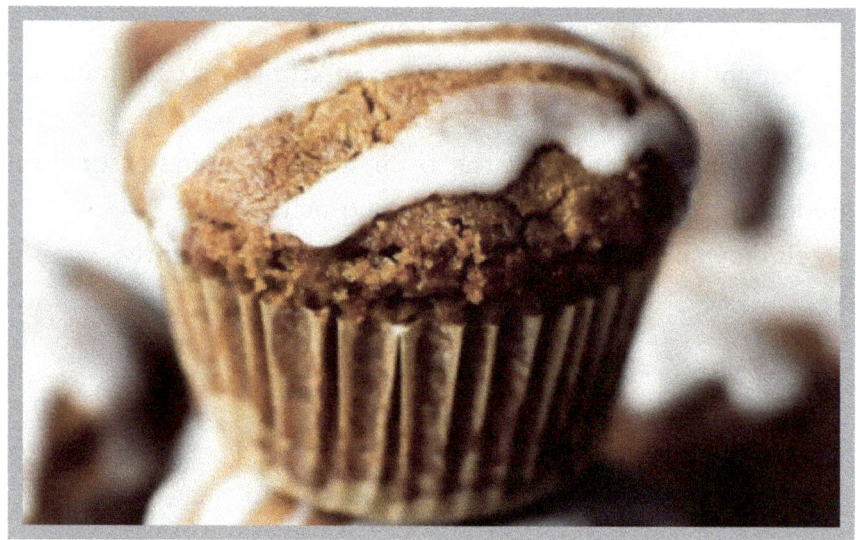

20 MINUTE

servings: 20

INGREDIENTS

1/2 cup almond flour

2 scoops of 32-34 grams of vanilla protein powder per scoop

1 teaspoon of baking powder

1 tablespoon of cinnamon

1/2 cup nut or seed butter of your choice: almond butter, peanut butter, sunflower seed butter, etc.

1/2 cup of pumpkin puree can be replaced with unsweetened applesauce, banana puree, or boiled sweet potato puree

1/2 cup coconut oil

For the icing on the cake

1/4 cup coconut butter

1/4 cup milk of your choice

1 tablespoon of granulated sweetener of your choice

2 teaspoons of lemon juice

manual

Preheat the oven to 350 Fahrenheit and then line out a 12-count muffin pan with muffin cups and set aside. You can also do this with a muffin tin.

In a large bowl, mix the dry ingredients and mix well. Add your wet ingredients and mix until fully incorporated.

Spread the cinnamon roll batter evenly on the muffin bowls. Bake for 10-15 minutes and check the 10 minute mark by inserting a skewer in the center and checking that it comes out clean. If so, the muffins are ready. Let it cool in the pan for 5 minutes before placing it on a rack to cool completely.

After cooling, glaze your cinnamon bun by combining all of the ingredients and stirring until everything is well mixed. Sprinkle the muffins on top and let harden.

Degree

For optimal freshness, low-carbohydrate cinnamon rolls

should be kept in the refrigerator. They can be stored in a covered container at room temperature, but must be used within 2 days.

To freeze muffins, wrap each serving individually.

nutrition

Serving size: 1 muffin | Calories: 112 kcal | Carbohydrates: 3 g | Protein: 5 g | Fat: 9 g | Potassium: 3 mg | Fiber: 2 g | Vitamin A: 50 IU | Vitamin C: 1.7 mg | Calcium: 10 mg | Iron: 0.2 mg | NET CARBOHYDRATES: 1 g

6

PALEO BANANA BREAD MUFFINS (GLUTEN-FREE, LOW-CARB)

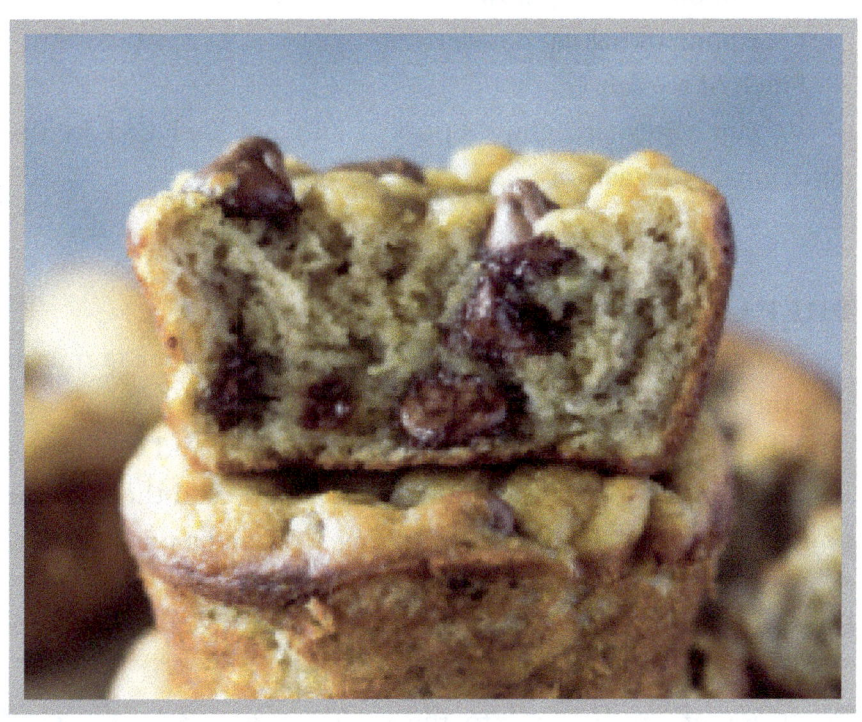

25 MINUTES

Servings: 12

INGREDIENTS

2 large eggs

2 cups mashed 3-4 medium-sized bananas

You can also use half a cup of peanut butter with almond butter

You can also use 1/4 cup buttered olive oil

1 teaspoon vanilla

You can also use 1/2 cup coconut flour, almond flour

1 tablespoon of cinnamon

1 teaspoon of baking powder

1 teaspoon of baking powder

Pinch of sea salt

1/2 cup chocolate chips optional and not included in the nutritional information

PREPARATION

Preheat the oven to 350 degrees. Grease or lay out 12 muffin tins; put aside.

Mix the eggs, bananas, almond butter, butter, and vanilla in a large bowl. Beat until everything is well mixed. Add the coconut flour, cinnamon, baking powder, baking soda, and a pinch of salt. Stir with a wooden spoon until everything is completely melted.

Pour 3/4 of the batter into the muffin bowls. Bake for 15-18 minutes or until golden brown. Let it cool for 10 minutes before removing it from the muffin pan. Store in the refrigerator for up to 4 days.

Degree

Recipe adapted from: Civilized Caveman Cooking

nutrition

Serving size: 1 muffin | Calories: 166 kcal | Carbohydrates: 14 g | Protein: 4 g | Fat: 11 g | Saturated fat: 4 g | Cholesterol: 37 mg | Sodium: 147 mg | Potassium: 256 mg | Fiber: 4 g | Sugar: 4 g | Vitamin A: 182 IU | Vitamin C: 3 mg | Calcium: 64 mg | Iron: 1 mg

7
LOW CARB MEDITERRANEAN EGG MUFFINS WITH HAM

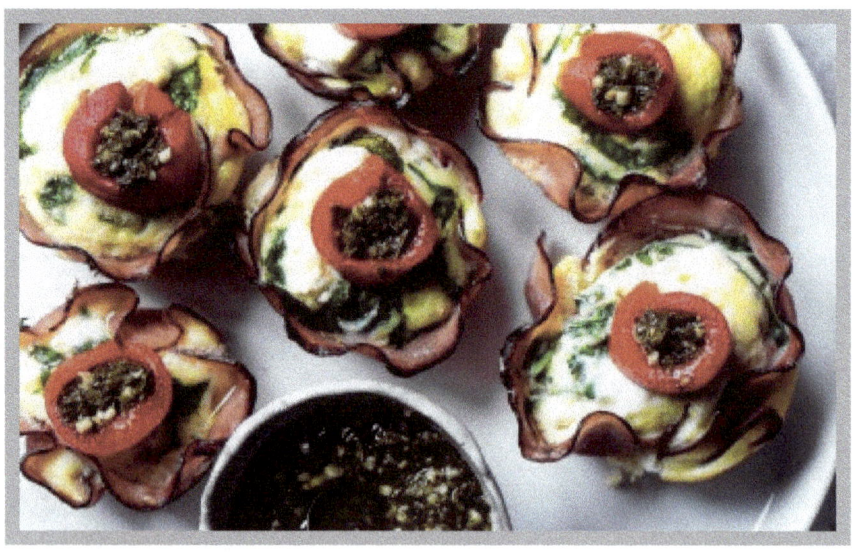

25 MINUTES
Servings 6

KETO CUPCAKE

. . .

INGREDIENTS

9 slices of raw ham thinly sliced
1/2 cup canned roasted red bell pepper, sliced + dressing
31/3 cup fresh spinach, chopped
41/4 cup feta cheese, crumbled
Large 5 large eggs
Salt InPinch
pinch of pepper
1/21 1/2 tablespoons pesto
Fresh basil to decorate

PREPARATION

Preheat the oven to 400 degrees. Spray GENERO muffin pan with cooking spray.

Line each muffin pan with 1.5 pieces of ham, making sure there are no holes for the egg mixture to explode.

Scoop a little toasted red bell pepper in the bottom of each muffin tin.

Put 1 tablespoon of chopped spinach on top of each red bell pepper.

Season the bell pepper and spinach with half a tablespoon of feta cheese.

In a medium bowl, whisk together the eggs, salt, and pepper. Spread the egg mixture evenly over the 6 muffin cups.

Cook for 15 to 17 minutes until the eggs are puffy and firm to the touch.

take off each cup from the muffin pan and garnish with 1/4 teaspoon pesto, roasted red pepper slices, and fresh basil.

Devour!

TIPS AND NOTES:

They are also very cold when you want to eat them for breakfast or a quick snack.

NUTRITIONAL INFORMATION:

Calories: 109 kcal (5%) Carbohydrates: 1.8 g (1%) Proteins: 9.3 g (19%) Fat: 6.7 g (10%) Saturated fat: 2.4 g (15%)) more times unsaturated fat: 0.9 g monounsaturated fat: 1.7 g cholesterol: 169 mg (56%) sodium: 423 mg (18%) potassium: 60 mg (2%) fiber: 1.8 g (8%) Sugar: 1.2 g (1%) Vitamin A: 500 IU (10)%) Vitamin C: 10.7 mg (13%) Calcium: 50 mg (5%) Iron: 0.9 mg (5%)

8

EIMUFFIN WITH PUMPKIN AND HAM

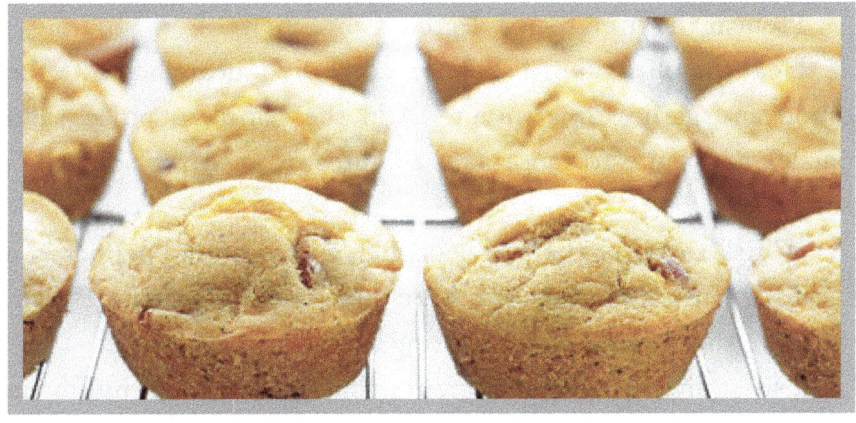

30 MINUTES
Servings 12

INGREDIENTS
1 tablespoon of olive oil

1/2 onion finely chopped
3 garlic cloves, minced
1 bell pepper, finely chopped
1 cup baby spinach, chopped
1/4 cup fresh parsley, minced
8 sizeable eggs
a quarter cup of coconut or nut milk
Season with salt and pepper to taste.
2 thinly sliced tiny zucchini
ham slices (12 slices)
Olive oil to coat the muffin tin

PREPARATION

Preheat the oven to 350 degrees Fahrenheit.

Heat the olive oil in a skillet over medium heat and sauté the onion and garlic for a minute. Add the paprika, spinach and parsley and sauté for another 2 minutes or until the spinach is soft.

Whisk together the eggs, coconut milk, salt and pepper in a bowl. Because when vegetables are done cooking, combine them with the sliced zucchini in a mixing bowl.

Using olive oil, grease a muffin tin and line each muffin tin with a slice of ham.

9
EGG MUFFINS

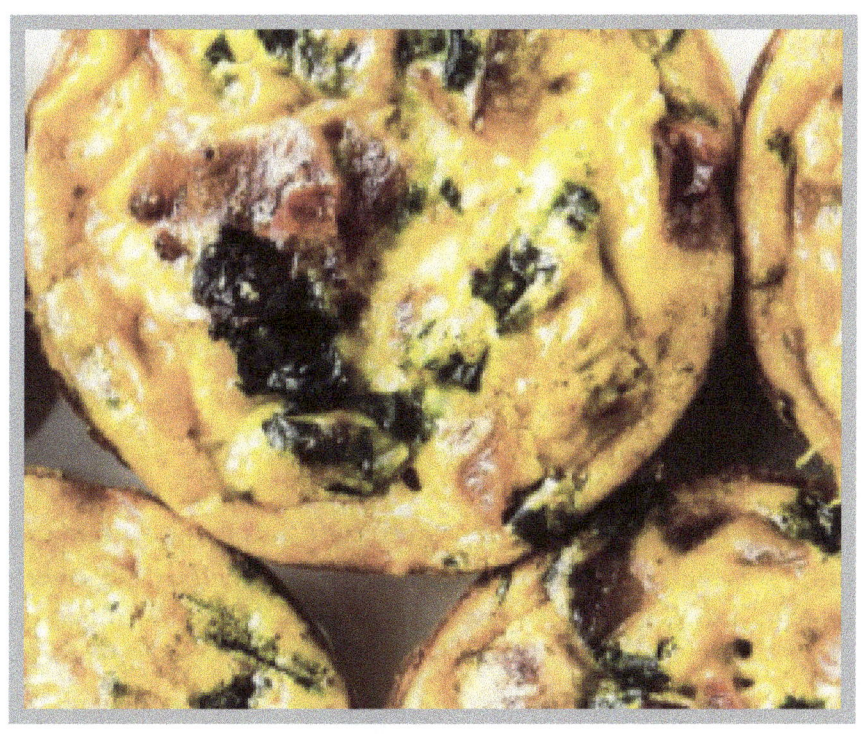

45 MINUTES

6 servings

INGREDIENTS

1 tablespoon of olive oil

8 ounces of sliced white mushrooms

Salt and freshly ground black pepper

100ml fresh spinach leaves and ¼ cup water OR 10 ounces frozen spinach, thawed

Eggs 6 lightly beaten eggs

6 ounces of crumbled feta cheese

PREHEAT THE OVEN to 375 ° F. Brush the muffin pan with non-stick cooking spray.

How to fry the mushrooms (optional, see notes):

In a large skillet, heat the oil over medium-high heat until it glows. Add the mushrooms and ¼ teaspoon of salt and cook until the mushrooms are tender and have released most of their liquid, about 5 minutes.

Using a slotted spoon, remove the mushrooms from the pan and transfer them to a large bowl. Leave the oil and remaining liquid in the pan.

How to use fresh spinach:

Add to the pan with water and saute for about 10 minutes until soft and wilted. Drain and place on a clean tea towel. Squeeze the towel and twist it to remove as much liquid as possible.

How to use frozen (thawed) spinach:

Fry in a pan for about 5 minutes until everything is heated

up. Drain them and place them on a clean cloth. Squeeze the towel and twist it to remove as much liquid as possible.

How to make egg muffins:

Put the spinach with mushrooms in the bowl. Add the eggs, cheese, ½ teaspoon of salt and ¼ teaspoon of pepper.

Spread the egg mixture evenly over 12 muffin bowls. Cook for about 25 minutes until the inserted toothpick is clean.

Allow to cool for a while before removing muffins from molds (egg cups should come out easily). Serve hot or at room temperature. Store leftovers in the refrigerator and consume them within 4 days.

How to freeze muffins:

Let cool and transfer in a single layer on a plate. Freeze for at least 30 minutes until solidified, then transfer to a freezer-safe bag. Freeze for up to 2 months.

How to reheat muffins:

Reheat directly from the freezer until heated, about 1 minute.

degrees

To save time, skip frying the mushrooms in oil. Slice very thinly and pour directly into raw muffin pans.

nutrition

Calories: 178 kcal

Carbohydrates: 4 g

Protein: 12 g

Fat: 13 g

Saturated fat: 6 g

Trans fat: 1 g

Cholesterol: 189 mg

Sodium: 418 mg

Potassium: 462 mg

Fiber: 1 g
Sugar: 2 g
Vitamin A: 4788 IU
Vitamin C: 14 mg
Calcium: 212 mg
Iron: 2 mg

10
KETO COFFEE CAKE MUFFIN

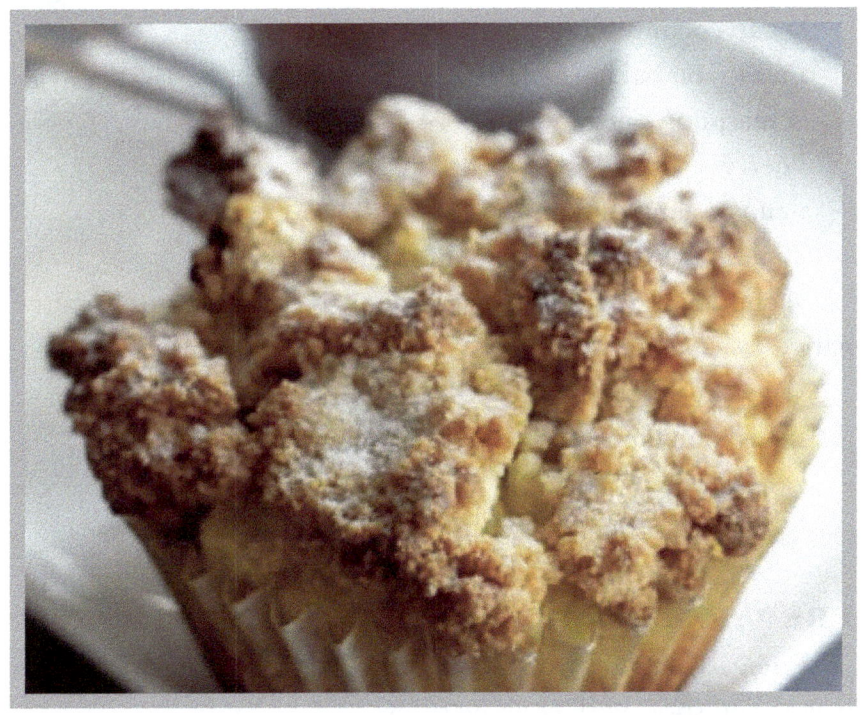

30 MINUTES
Servings 12

INGREDIENTS

Mass:
Tables 2 tablespoons soft butter
200g soft cream cheese
⅓ Cup of Joy Filled Eats Sweetener (or see alternatives in recipe notes)
4 eggs
Teas 2 teaspoons vanilla
½ cup unsweetened vanilla almond milk
1 cup of almond flour
½ cup coconut flour
1 teaspoon baking soda
¼ teaspoon salt
Poetry:
1 cup of almond flour
Tables 2 tablespoons coconut flour
¼ cup Joy Filled Eats sweetener (or see recipe notes for alternatives)
¼ cup butter, softened
1 teaspoon cinnamon
½ teaspoon molasses *** (optional)

PREPARATION

Preheat oven to 350. Line a standard muffin tin with paper inserts and spray with cooking spray.

Combine all of the dough ingredients in a food processor. Mix well. Spread on prepared muffin pan.

Combine garnished ingredients in food processor and blend until crumbs form. Sprinkle over the dough.

Bake until golden brown for 20-25 minutes. If the crumb topping gets too dark, cover it with aluminum foil for the last 5 minutes.

Observations

I get a bunch of comments from my low carb readers about using molasses. I use it for the flavor, not the sweetness. 5 grams of carbohydrates are contained in one teaspoon of molasses. Half a teaspoon is divided by 12 servings in this recipe. Molasses contains less than 0.25 grams of carbohydrates. You can miss it if you want.

Suggestions for sweeteners:

In my recipes, I use a custom blend of xylitol, erythritol, and stevia. It has twice the sweetness of sugar. Trim Healthy Mama Gentle Sweet and Truvia are close.

To add Pyure or Trim Healthy Mama Super Sweet, use half the amount of sweetener needed.

Substitutions work in most recipes. They may not work in candies like caramel.

NUTRITION

Serving size: 1 muffin | Calories: 222 | Carbohydrates: 9 g |

Proteins: 7 g | Fat: 18 g | Saturated fat: 6 g | Cholesterol: 72 mg | Sodium: 156 mg | Potassium: 73 mg | Fiber: 4 g | Sugar: 1 g | Vitamin A: 290 IU | Calcium: 86 mg | Iron: 1.2 mg

LOW CARB ALMOND AND LEMON FLOUR MUFFINS FILLED WITH BLACKBERRIES

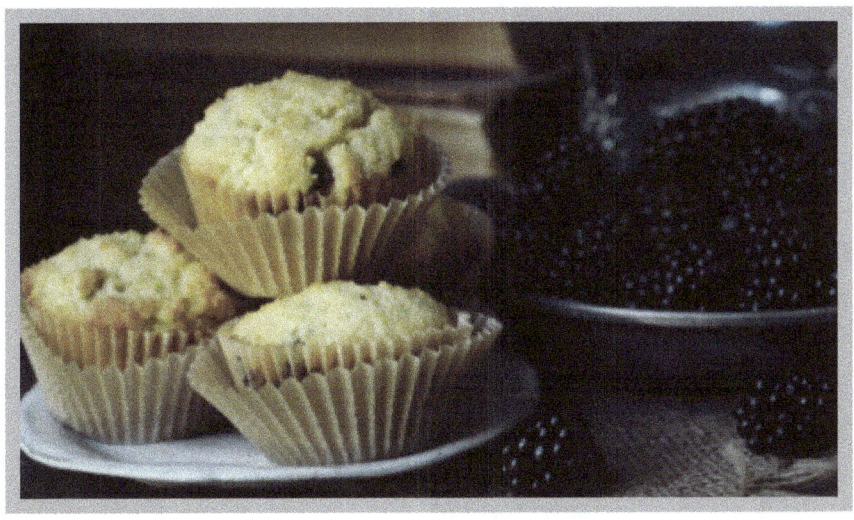

45 MINUTES

Servings 12

. . .

INGREDIENTS

For the blackberry filling:

3 tablespoons granular stevia / erythritol (pyure) blend

1/4 teaspoon of xanthan gum

2 tablespoons of water

1 tablespoon of lemon juice

1 cup of fresh or frozen blackberries

For the muffin batter:

2 and h cups super fine almond flour

3/4 cup granular stevia / erythritol blend

1 teaspoon of fresh lemon zest

1/2 teaspoon of sea salt

1 teaspoon of grain-free baking powder

4 large eggs

1/4 cup original flavored unsweetened almond milk

1/4 cup melted butter, ghee, or coconut oil

1 teaspoon of vanilla extract

1/2 teaspoon of lemon extract

PREPARATION

For the blackberry filling:

In a 1 1/2 liter saucepan, mix the granulated sweetener and xanthan gum. Add the water and lemon juice one tablespoon at a time, mixing between each addition.

LEMON MUFFINS With Low Carb Almond Flour Filled With Blackberries, Ready Berries.

Add the blackberries to the mix. Preheat the skillet to

medium-low. Get the mixture to a boil, constantly stirring. Reduce the temperature.

Blackberry muffins made with low-carb lemon and almond flour, with blackberries added for the filling.

Cook for about 10 minutes over low heat, stirring regularly, until the berries have broken down and a thick jam syrup has formed. take off the pan from the heat and set aside to cool.

Low carb muffins with lemon and almond flour, filled with blackberries and blackberries

For the muffin batter:
Preheat the oven to 350° Fahrenheit. Prepare a muffin pan by lining it with muffin wrappers.

In a medium bowl, combine the almond flour, granulated sweetener, lemon zest, sea salt, and baking powder.

Lemon Almond Flour Stuffed With Blackberry Low Carb Muffins - Dry Ingredients.

Combine the eggs, almond milk, vanilla extract, and lemon extract in a small mixing bowl. While you whisk, drizzle in the sugar.

. . .

Low-carb muffins made with lemon and almond flour and blackberries, with ready-to-mix liquid ingredients.

Slowly insert liquid ingredients to the dry ingredients while stirring.

Low carb lemon and almond flour muffin batter filled with blackberries

Pour the batter into the prepared muffin pans to fill about 1/3 full. Use clean fingers or a spoon to make a hollow in the batter in the cups.

Low carb lemon and almond flour muffins filled with blackberries - ready for blackberry filling.

Add a tablespoon of frozen blackberry jam to each well and distribute it evenly between the cups.

Low-carb lemon and almond flour muffins filled with blackberries that add blackberry filling.

Cover the blackberry jam with the rest of the batter until each cup is about 2/3 full. Spread the batter over the edges of the bowls to cover as much of the jam as possible. If the cups are just over 2/3 full after the batter is used up, that's fine.

. . .

Low-carb lemon and almond flour muffins filled with blackberries, ready to bake

do Baking in the preheated oven for 25-30 minutes or until the top pops out again when you touch it lightly.

Low-carb almond flour lemon muffins filled with freshly baked blackberries

Cool extra in an airtight container. If desired, they can also be frozen.

Notes on the recipe
For muffins:

Total carbohydrates (g): 4

Dietary fiber (g): 3

Net carbohydrates: 1 gram

EGG MUFFIN FOR BREAKFAST 3 WAYS

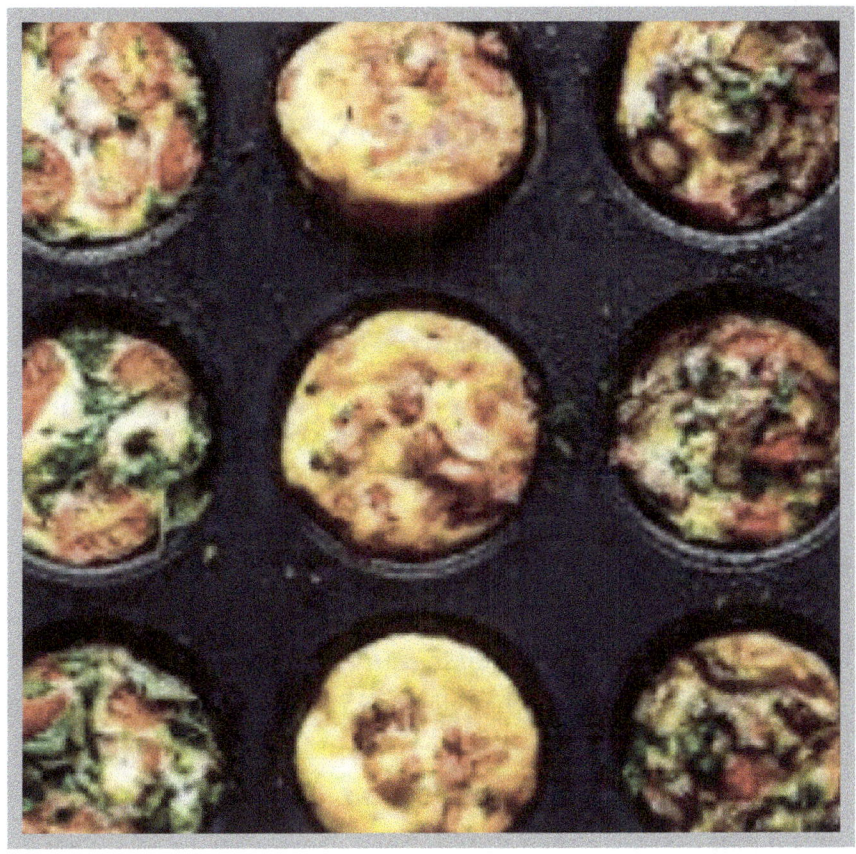

35 MINUTES

Server 12

INGREDIENTS

a dozen big eggs

2 tablespoons red, white, or yellow / brown onion, finely chopped

Season with salt and pepper to taste.

SPINACH TOMATO MOZZARELLA:

1/4 cup fresh spinach, roughly chopped

8 cherry tomatoes or cherry tomatoes, halved
1/4 cup mozzarella grated
CHEDDAR bacon:
1/4 cup cooked bacon, chopped
1/4 cup shredded cheddar cheese
PEPPER MUSHROOMS WITH GARLIC:
1/4 cup sliced brown mushrooms
1/4 cup red bell pepper (paprika), diced
1 tablespoon minced fresh parsley
1/4 teaspoon garlic powder or 1/3 teaspoon minced garlic

PREPARATION

Preheat oven to 350 ° F to 180 ° C. Lightly spray a 12-cup muffin pan with nonstick cooking spray.

In a large bowl, beat the eggs and onion. Spice with salt and pepper.

Add the egg mixture in half to each pan of a greased muffin pan.

Divide the three topping combinations into 4 muffin cups each.

Cook for 15 to 20 minutes until solid.

Let cool slightly, then serve OR refrigerate in an airtight container for up to 4 days and reheat to serve.

Enjoy!

NUTRITION

Calories: 82kcal | Carbohydrates: 1 g | Proteins: 6 g | Fat: 5 g | Saturated fat: 2 g | Cholesterol: 168 mg | Sodium: 97 mg | Potassium: 103 mg | Vitamin A: 555 IU | Vitamin C: 6.3 mg | Calcium: 55 mg | Iron: 0.8 mg

13

CHOCOLATE PEANUT BUTTER MUFFINS

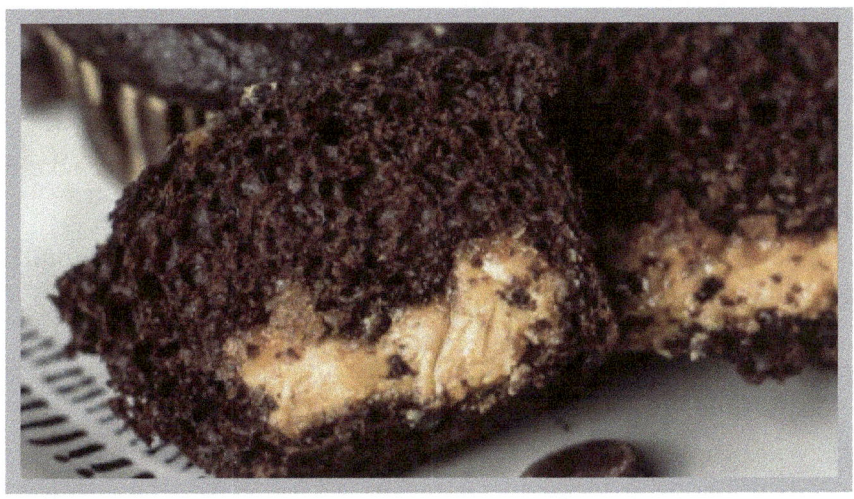

25 MINUTES
Servings 6

INGREDIENTS

1 cup of almond flour

1/2 cup of this nourished erythritol sweetener

1 teaspoon baking powder

1 pinch of salt

1/3 cup peanut butter

1/3 cup almond milk

2 large eggs

1/2 cup cacao nibs (or unsweetened chocolate chips)

PREPARATION

Pre-heat oven to 350 degrees F and mix together all of the dry ingredients (except the cocoa beans) in a big mixing bowl.

Combine the peanut butter and almond milk in a mixing dish.

Add 1 egg at a time, mixing well after each addition.

Add the unsweetened chocolate nuggets or cocoa nuggets.

Cooking spray a muffin tin and roll out the batter to make 6 big muffins.

Bake for 20-30 minutes and cool completely. Have fun with some butter or a splash of unsweetened maple syrup.

14
KETO CARROT CAKE MUFFINS

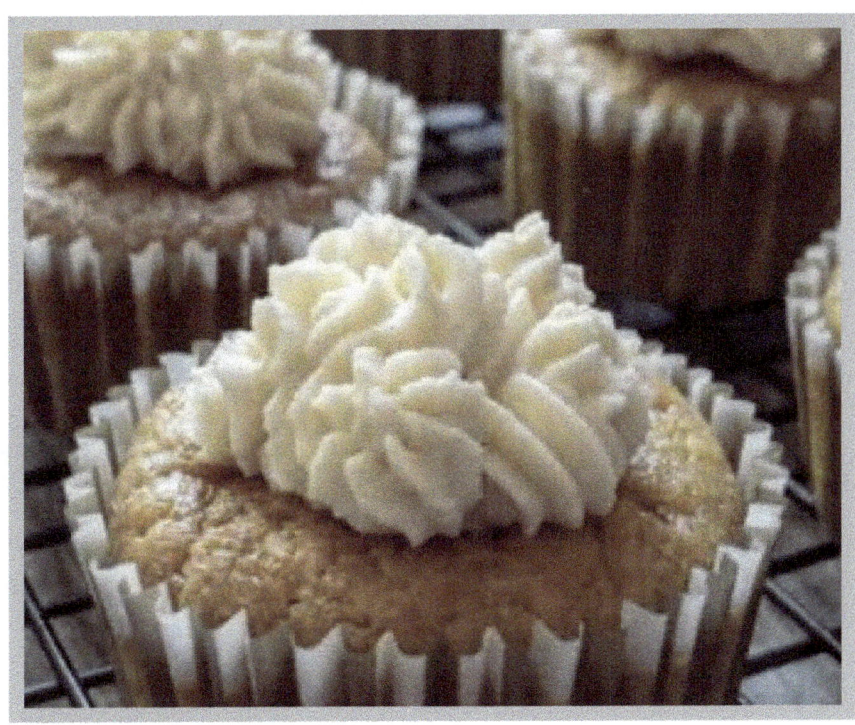

1 HOUR 5 minutes
Servings 4

INGREDIENTS
Muffin
1 cup of almond flour
1/2 cup lakanto monk fruit
1 teaspoon of baking powder
1 teaspoon of cinnamon
1/2 teaspoon salt
3/4 cup olive oil
2 beaten eggs
3 small carrots, grated (about 1 / 2-3 / 4 cup, grated)
cream
4 ounces of cream cheese at room temperature
2 tablespoons of butter at room temperature
1/4 cup Lakanto monk fruit powder
2 tablespoons heavy whipped cream
1/2 teaspoon vanilla extract
1/4 teaspoon almond extract
4 drops of liquid stevia

PREPARATION
CAKE:

PREHEAT THE OVEN to 350 degrees.

. . .

PLACE the muffin bowls in the baking tray (12).

COMBINE THE ALMOND FLOUR, monk fruit, baking powder, cinnamon, and salt in a large mixing bowl. Using a spatula or a brush, thoroughly combine the ingredients.

WITH THE WHISK, blend the olive oil, eggs, and grated carrots. Don't overmix; about 15-30 seconds should suffice!
 Also pour the batter into the muffin tins.

COOK for 40-45 minutes or until centered.

SET ASIDE TO COOL.

CREAM

USING A CLEAN WHISK, combine the butter and cream cheese in a medium mixing bowl.

CONTINUE TO BEAT in the monk fruit, heavy cream, vanilla, almonds, and stevia until well combined.

. . .

STORE FROST-CHILLED CUPCAKES and in an airtight container in the refrigerator!

15
LOW CARB KETO CHOCOLATE MUFFINS

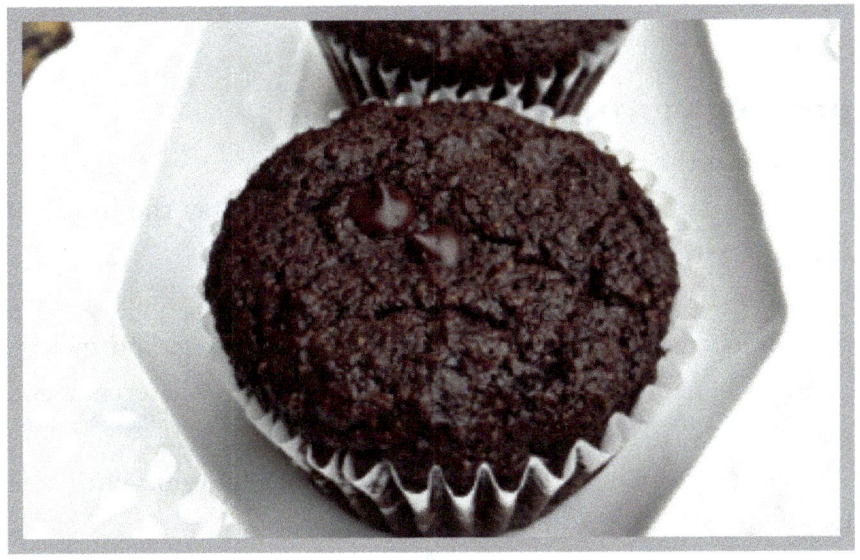

40 MINUTES
Servings: 9

. . .

INGREDIENTS

1/2 cup coconut flour
3/4 teaspoon baking powder
2 tablespoons of cocoa powder
1/2 teaspoon salt
1 teaspoon of cinnamon
1/2 teaspoon nutmeg
3 large eggs
2/3 cup granulated sweetener
2 teaspoons of vanilla extract
1 tablespoon of oil
1 cup wrapped shredded zucchini
1/4 cup of heavy cream
1/3 cup unsweetened chocolate chips

PREPARATION

Preheat the oven to 350F

Line a 12-cup pan with 9 muffin tins and spray the inside of the cups with cooking spray.

allow In a medium bowl, combine coconut flour, baking powder, cocoa powder, salt, cinnamon, sweetener, and nutmeg.

In a separate bowl, mix the eggs, vanilla, oil, cream and zucchini.

Add the wet ingredients to the dry ones and mix until well blended. Work in the chocolate chips.

Pour the batter into the muffin pans and bake for 30 minutes or until the toothpick is clean.

Take off the oven and let cool in a pan.

These keto chocolate muffins should be refrigerated for up to 1 week or see instructions on freezing.

16

CINNAMON, FLAX AND WALNUT MUFFINS

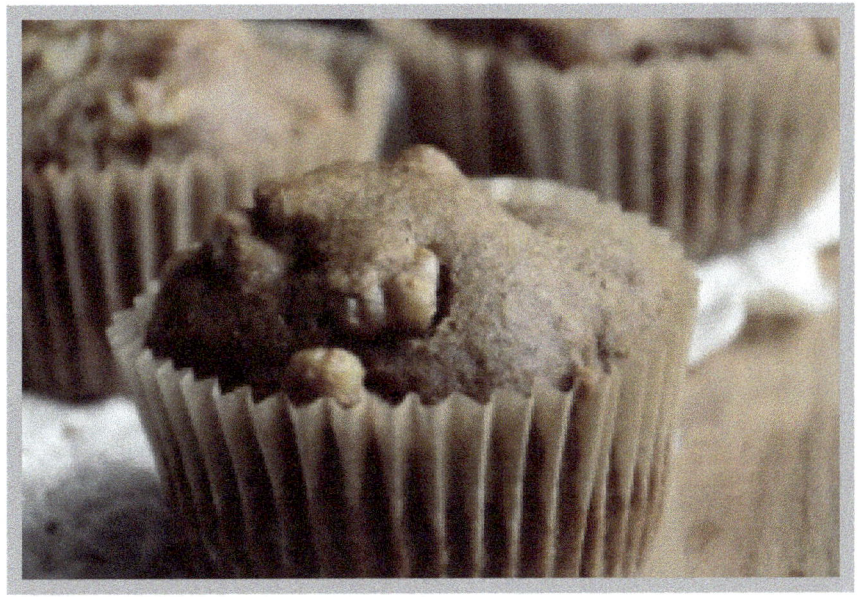

30 MINUTES
Servings 12

. . .

INGREDIENTS

Buy 1 cup of ground golden flaxseed or pre-ground flaxseed meal

4 grass eggs

1/2 cup avocado oil or any oil

1/2 cup granulated sweetener (maple sugar, erythritol, lakanto, coconut sugar)

1/4 cup coconut flour

2 teaspoons vanilla extract

2 teaspoons cinnamon

1 teaspoon lemon juice

1/2 teaspoon baking powder

A pinch of sea salt

1 cup of chopped walnuts

PREPARATION

Preheat to 325 * F.

If you start with whole golden flax seeds, grind them in a coffee grinder and then measure 1 cup.

Note: I like to use golden flax seeds because I find the flavor milder than dark brown flax seeds, but any colored flax will work.

In a bowl, mix the ingredients in the order shown. You can use an electric mixer if you want, but be sure to add the walnuts last after using a mixer.

Bake at 325 * F for 18-22 minutes. I recommend using muffins to prevent sticking and to make the muffins more "portable."

Nutrition information estimated using myfitnesspal 1 muffin per serving, based on a total of 12 muffins. The following data is based on the use of a sugar alcohol for sweetening. If you use coconut sugar, add 8 carbs and 30 calories per muffin.

CALORIES: 219
  Total fat: 20 grams
  Total carbohydrates: 6 grams
  Dietary fiber: 4 grams
  Sugar: 1 gram
  Protein: 6 grams

MUFFIN KETO - CLASSIC "SUGAR" DONUT WITH CINNAMON

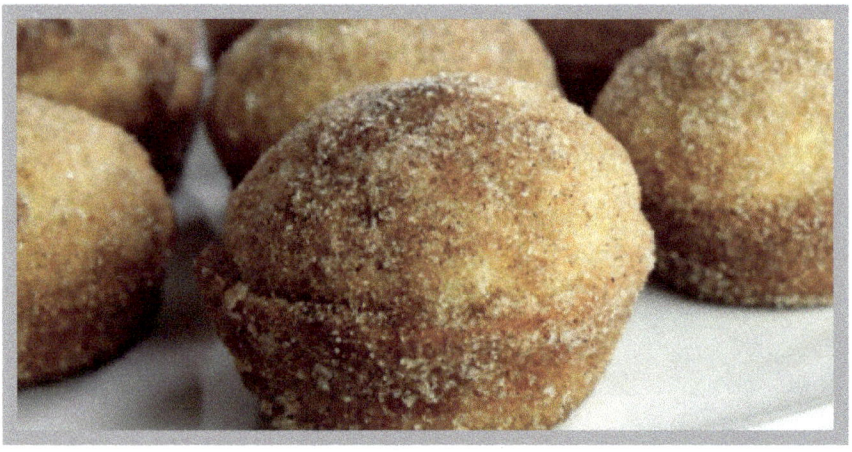

30 MINUTES
Servings 4

INGREDIENTS

½ cup of cream

KETO CUPCAKE

5 tablespoons butter, softened

2 large eggs

1 teaspoon vanilla

½ cup powdered sweetener, 20% discount at Lakanto with code MELISSA20

1 ½ cup of blanched almond flour

2 tablespoons psyllium husk powder

2 teaspoons of baking soda

1/2 teaspoon of nutmeg

1/2 teaspoon ginger

1/4 teaspoon allspice

FOR THE COVER:

2 tablespoons melted butter

1 teaspoon cinnamon

¼ cup granulated sweetener

PREPARATION

Preheat oven to 350. Line a muffin tin with aluminum foil.

Using an electric mixer, beat the buttercream, sweetener, and vanilla until smooth in a medium dish. Combine the eggs and milk in a mixing bowl.

Combine all dry ingredients in a separate dish (except filling ingredients). Slowly add to the wet ingredients and continue to combine using an electric mixer.

In - muffin cup, put a tablespoon.

you are to Bake for 18-20 minutes, or until golden brown and crisp around the edges.

Allow it to cool fully before using.

Brush the finished muffins with butter, roll in the cinnamon and sweetener mixture. To serve!

NUTRITIONAL INFORMATION: YIELD: 12 SERVING SIZE: 1

Amount per serving: CALORIES: 200 TOTAL FAT: 18 g TRANSFAT: 0 g CARBON HYDRATES: 5 g NET CARBON HYDRATE: 2 g FIBERS: 3 g ALCOHOLIC SUGAR: 0 g PROTEIN: 5 g

18

KETO CHEDDAR AND BROCCOLI MUFFINS

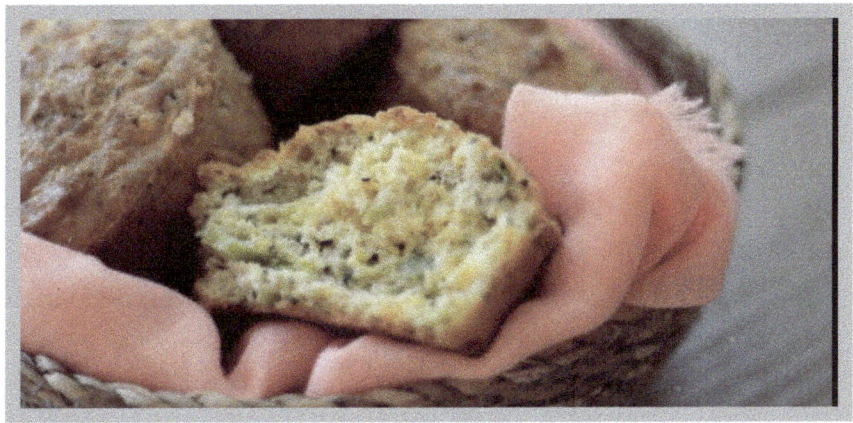

40 min
 Servings 4

INGREDIENTS
 Raw egg

Big 3
Thick cream
¼ cup of salted butter
2 tbsp
Unprepared frozen broccoli
5 oz
Cheddar cheese
½ cup of grated cheese
Salt
¼ teaspoon of ground black pepper
⅛ teaspoon of almond flour
1 cup of baking soda
½ tsp

PREPARATION

Cooking time 40 min

Preheat the oven to 350 degrees. blend the eggs and cream in a bowl. Melt the butter and stir in 3-4 additions so that the butter does not boil the egg.

THAWING broccoli finely chopped and whipped with cheddar cheese. Also add the salt and pepper.

FINALLY ADD the remaining almond flour and baking powder.

Pour the batter into a 6-carat muffin pan that has been lightly sprayed with pan spray with no paper liner required.

Bake the pan for 20 minutes. Then reduce the oven temperature to 325 degrees and bake for another 10 minutes. allow it cool for 5 minutes before removing it from the pan.

19

MUFFINS WITH KETO RASPBERRIES AND WHITE CHOCOLATE

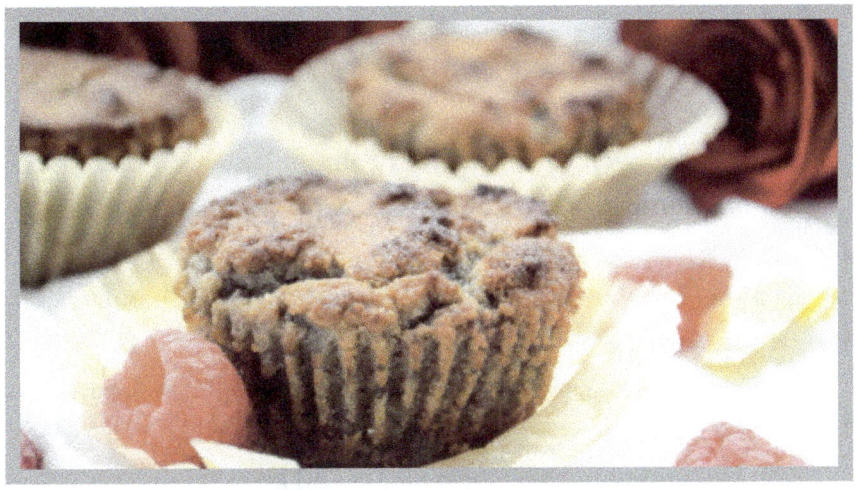

28 MINUTES
 Servings 18

. . .

INGREDIENTS

Wet Ingredients:

1/2 cup cocoa, melted but not hot

1/2 cup Dietz sweet or coconut sugar - not ketogenic

4 hard-boiled eggs

1/4 cup whole coconut milk

1 teaspoon vanilla extract

Dry ingredients:

2-1/2 cups of superfine almond flour

1/4 cup grass-fed collagen

2 tablespoons of coconut flour

1-1/4 teaspoons of baking soda

1 teaspoon of baking powder

1 cup finely chopped frozen raspberries

PREPARATION

Preheat the oven to 350 degrees Fahrenheit.

Line a muffin pan with unbleached baking paper or silicone muffin.

In a medium bowl, combine all of the dry ingredients except the frozen raspberries. Put aside.

In the bowl of a food processor, combine the melted cocoa butter and sweetener.

Add the remaining wet ingredients and keep mixing.

Add the dry ingredients while the blender is running. When it is well mixed, turn off the mixer.

Work in the frozen raspberries.

Pour about 2 tablespoons of muffin batter into each of the muffin holes.

Bake for 20 to 22 minutes or until golden brown.

Remove from oven and allow to cool.

keep it in an airtight container inside refrigerator.

20
SUPER TENDER AND MOIST KETO PUMPKIN CUPCAKES

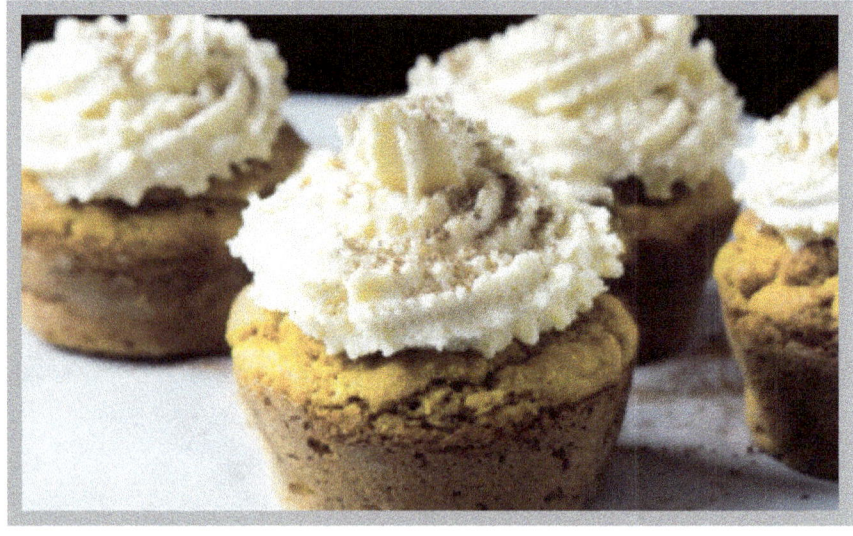

30 MINUTES
Servings 6

. . .

INGREDIENTS

For the keto pumpkin cupcakes:

64 g of almond flour

21 g coconut flour

1/2 teaspoon xanthan gum

1 teaspoon baking powder

1/4 teaspoon baking powder

1 half teaspoons homemade pumpkin pie spice

1/4 teaspoon kosher salt

2 eggs lightly beaten

2-3 tablespoons of piure

1 teaspoon vanilla extract

1 teaspoon apple cider vinegar

25g coconut oil, melted

110 g canned pumpkin puree

60 ml of almond milk

2 tablespoons of chopped walnuts

To glaze

1/2 batch of cream cheese butter frosting optional

Homemade Pumpkin Pie Spices for Sprinkles

PREPARATION

Preheat the oven to 180 ° C.

Muffin tin with butter and flour. Put aside.

Whisk together the almond flour, coconut flour, xanthan gum, baking powder, pumpkin pie spice, and salt in a medium mixing bowl. Remove from the equation.

Combine the eggs and piura in a big mixing bowl. whisk the mixture for 2 minutes, or until light and fluffy, with an electric mixer. In a mixing bowl, whisk together the vanilla extract, vinegar, coconut oil, and pumpkin puree until smooth. Alternate adding the almond milk and the dry flour mixture. After you've finished working, fold in the walnuts. Combine the eggs and piura in a big mixing bowl. whisk the mixture for 2 minutes, or until light and fluffy, with an electric mixer. Combine the vanilla extract, vinegar, coconut oil, and pumpkin puree in a mixing bowl and beat until smooth. Alternate incorporating the dry flour mixture and the almond milk. Fold in the walnuts after you've finished working.

Distribute batter evenly in skillet. Cook for 18-20 minutes (at 15, cover with aluminum foil) until golden brown and a toothpick inserted comes out clean.

Let cool in the pan for 15 minutes before removing and place on a wire rack to cool completely before frosting.

Make the buttercream cheese frosting while the cakes cool. And away the frost!

make sure it covered and refrigerated for up to 3 days, although we're pretty sure they'll be gone by then.

OBSERVATIONS

* When choosing a sweetener for stevia, we like Pyure best. We think it is quite sweet (although it is technically only twice as sweet as sugar). So keep adding them one by one to test! 2 tablespoons are enough, especially if it is with glaze. However, you are free to raise the number to three.

Try 3-5 scoops of Swerve if you're using it!

Please keep in mind that the nutritional information is for ketogenic pumpkin cupcakes only. However, keep in mind the one serving of our Butter

NUTRITION

Calories: 154 kcal | Carbohydrates: 6 g | Proteins: 4 g | Fat

21
LOW CARB STRAWBERRY LEMONADE MUFFINS

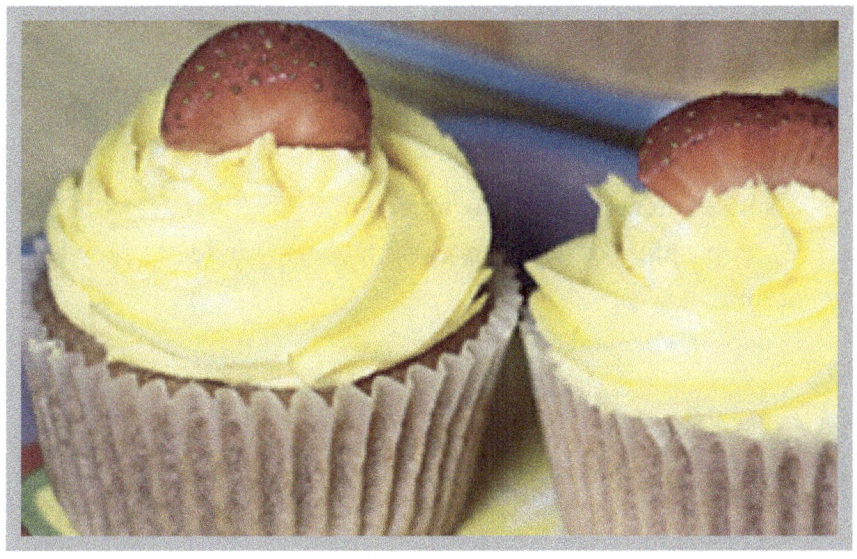

1 HOUR
Servings 12

· · ·

INGREDIENTS

Muffin:

2 1/3 cups almond flour

¾ Dodge the sweetener cup

quarter cup unflavored whey protein powder (or egg white protein powder)

2 teaspoons of baking soda

½ teaspoon of salt

3 large eggs

½ cup butter, melted

Zest of 1 lemon

¼ cup fresh lemon juice

1 teaspoon lemon extract

¼ cup extra water if needed

Nail polish:

6 ounces frozen strawberries, thawed

2 tablespoons fresh lemon juice

1/2 cup butter, softened

4 ounces cream cheese, softened

½ cup plus 2 tablespoons Swerve divided powdered sweetener

½ cup of whipped cream

PREPARATION

muffin

start by Preheating oven to 350F and line a muffin pan with parchment paper or silicone film.

In a large bowl, combine the almond flour, sweetener, protein powder, baking powder, and salt. Add the eggs, melted butter, lemon zest, lemon juice, lemon extract, and water and mix until smooth. put more water if the dough is too thick.

Spread over prepared muffin tins and smooth out the tips. Cook for 25-30 minutes, until it is a nice golden brown color and to the touch. Remove and let cool completely.

Nail polish

Combine the strawberries and lemon juice in a blender or food processor. Put aside.

Beat cream cheese and butter until smooth. Mix in ½ cup of the powdered sweetener, then blend in the strawberry puree until smooth.

In another bowl, beat the whipped cream with the remaining 2 tablespoons of powdered sweetener until the tips are very hard.

Gently stir in the cream cheese mixture and the whipped cream until there are no more stripes. Place them on the cooled cupcakes and let them sit in the refrigerator for at least 1 hour.

nutrition

Serving size: 1 cupcake | Calories: 366 kcal | Carbohydrates: 7.5 g | Proteins: 9.2 g | Fat: 32.6 g | Fiber: 2.7 g

22

GLUTEN-FREE AND KETOGENIC GINGERBREAD CUPCAKES

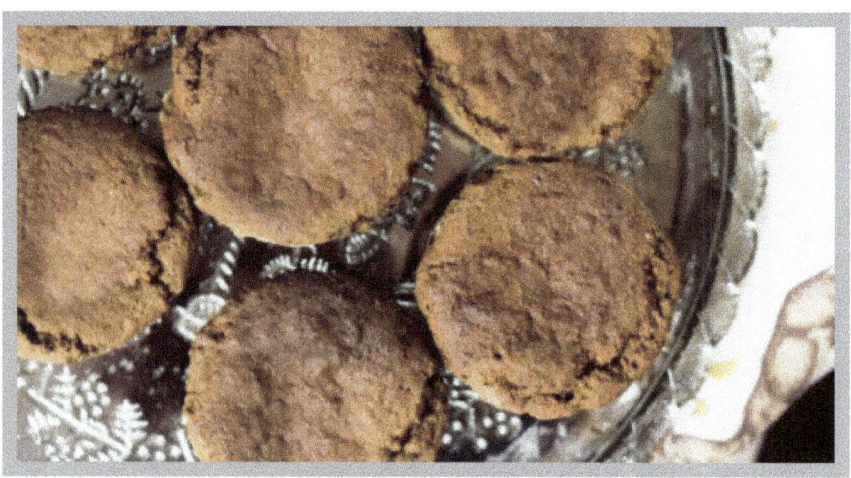

30 MINUTES
Servings 6

INGREDIENTS

For the keto gingerbread cupcakes

64 g almond flour

21 g coconut flour

1 tablespoon psyllium husk

1/2 teaspoon of xanthan gum or 2 teaspoons of ground flaxseed

1/2 teaspoon baking powder

1/2 teaspoon baking powder

1/4 teaspoon kosher salt

1 teaspoon of ground ginger

1 teaspoon ground cinnamon

1/4 teaspoon freshly grated nutmeg

1/8 teaspoon ground cloves

Pinch of freshly ground black pepper

2 egg yolks and the divided egg white

1/3-1/2 cup golden erythritol to taste (I use 1/3 cup)

1-2 teaspoons of black cocoa molasses completely optional

1 teaspoon apple cider vinegar

57 g grass-fed unsalted fat or coconut oil (melted and chilled)

60 ml of water

For the lemon curd glaze

1/2 batch of keto buttercream icing

PREPARATION

Set the oven to 180 degrees Celsius. Using fat and flour, grease a muffin tin (with coconut flour).

Inside a medium mixing bowl, put the almond flour, coconut flour, psyllium husk, xanthan gum, baking powder, salt, and spices. Take it out of the equation.

Set aside the egg whites after beating them until soft peaks emerge.

Lightly and loosely beat the egg yolks with the sweetener in a big mixing bowl with an electric mixer on medium speed for 1-3 minutes.

Combine the molasses (optional), vinegar, and melted butter in a mixing bowl. Slowly whisk in the flour mixture, alternating with water, until thoroughly mixed.

Work the egg white into the dough slowly and carefully. The batter is thick at first, but as soon as you stir it, it loosens up. Note that keto pie crusts are more like cookie dough than can actually be poured (don't worry!).

put the batter inside the prepared muffin pan and match the top to the back of a damp spoon (or fingertips).Bake for 18-20 minutes (at 15, cover with foil) until golden brown and an inserted toothpick clean.

Let it cool in the pan for 15 minutes before taking it out of the oven, and if it's glazed, chill completely on a rack. Remember, it's best to enjoy them completely cold when the flavors have had a chance to blend. And the next day they are MUCH better when all the spices are set.

While the gingerbread cupcakes are cooling, make the lemon buttercream frosting by adding the zest of a lemon to our buttercream frosting. Alternatively, you can also make a cinnamon glaze! (Add about 1 teaspoon of cinnamon).

Store in an airtight container without icing for up to 3 days, although I'm pretty sure they will go away much sooner

23
KETO COCONUT FLOUR CUPCAKES

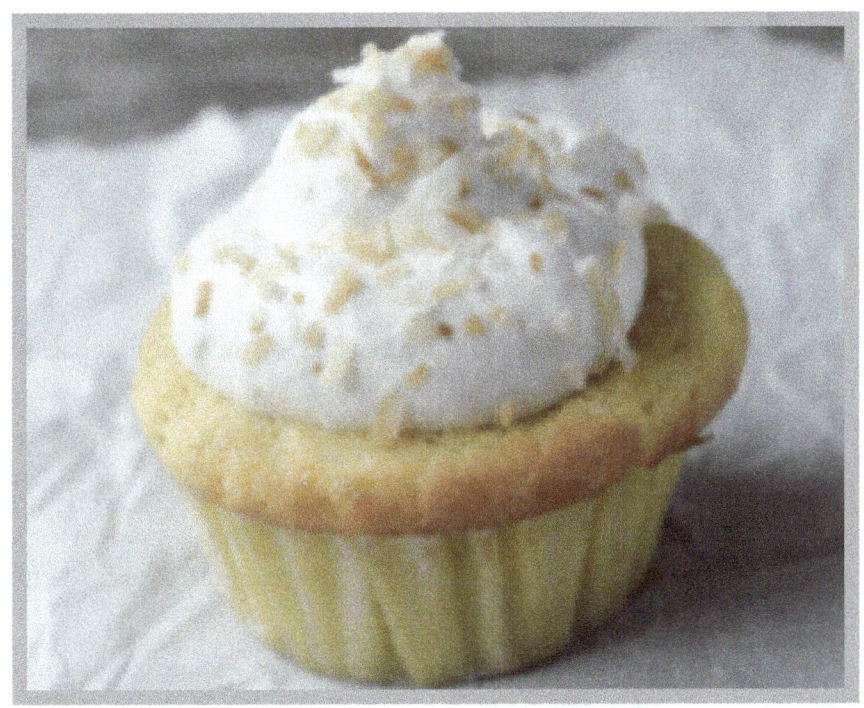

50 MINUTES

Serving 4

INGREDIENTS

2/3 cups coconut flour

1/2 cup of butter

1 cup erythritol

2 teaspoons baking powder

1 teaspoon vanilla extract

1 cup of coconut cream

2 ounces cream cheese

4 large eggs

PREPARATION

Preheat the oven to 350 degrees Fahrenheit.

Line cupcake pan with sleeve or generously brush 12 individual cups with butter

Combine the coconut flour and baking powder in a large bowl and set aside.

Cut the butter into several squares and put it in a separate bowl, add the cream cheese

Cook the butter and cream cheese in the microwave for 30 seconds. Be careful not to burn the cream cheese. Mix these wet ingredients until well combined.

Add the erythritol, vanilla extract, and coconut cream to the butter and cream cheese mixture. Mix well.

Pour the wet ingredients into a large bowl with coconut flour and baking powder. Mix well.

Add the eggs to the batter. Mix well.

Pour the batter into a cake pan, place in the oven and bake for 35 minutes, or until a toothpick in the cake is clean.

For best results, allow cake to cool completely for at least 2 hours, preferably overnight. If you remove it too soon, it may fall apart a bit.

Observations

Coconut cream is very similar to coconut milk. If you want, you can cool the coconut milk to separate the cream from the water and use it in this recipe. Separation can be done in just 30 minutes.

EVERY STOVE IS DIFFERENT. Keep an eye on your cake and check it out while it bakes.

IF THE CAKE seems too moist, return it to the oven at 5 minute intervals until it is cooked through. It should bounce when touched lightly, but may wobble slightly. This is typical for coconut flour desserts until completely cold.

24
MINT CHOCOLATE CUPCAKES (KETO, PALEO)

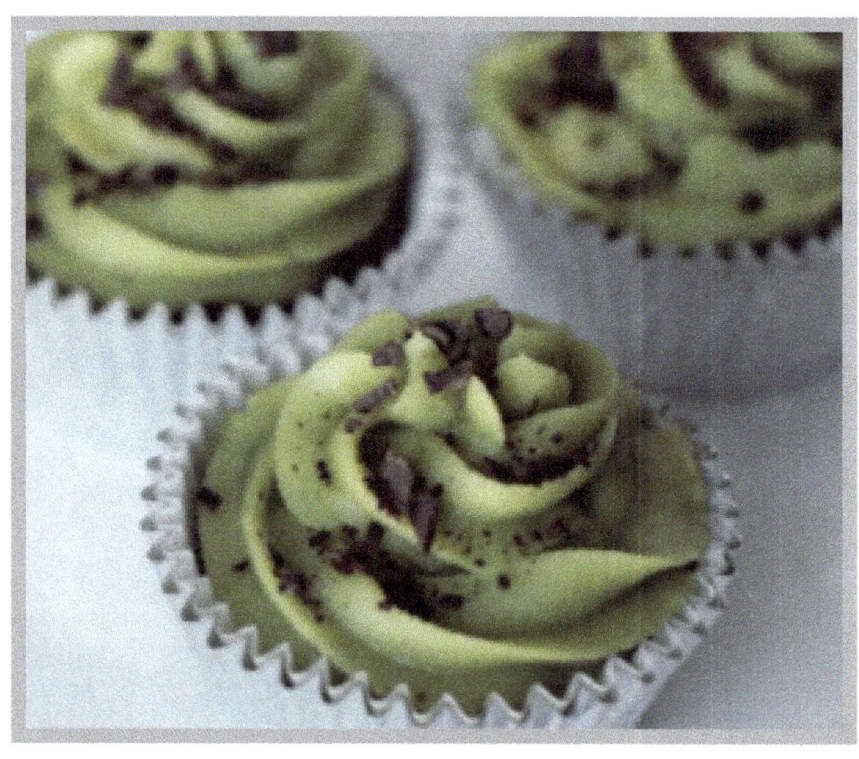

KETO CUPCAKE

45 MINUTES

Servings 8

INGREDIENTS

Chocolate cupcakes (dairy-free)

¾ cup of warm coconut butter

⅔ Cup sweetener of your choice Monkfruit sweetener (see link below in recipe notes or the most popular low carb sweetener) works for keto, honey for GAPS / paleo, coconut sugar / maple syrup for paleo too

½ cup of melted hot coconut oil or other liquid fat: melted warm butter / ghee, melted warm lard, avocado oil

½ cup of Fairtrade cocoa powder, see recipe notes for the link to good cocoa

2 eggs at room temperature (not cold); You can do this by placing cold eggs in a glass of hot water for 30 minutes.

¼ cup coconut flour

¼ cup whole, warm (not cold) coconut milk or raw whole milk if tolerated

1 teaspoon of gelatin see link in recipe notes

1 teaspoon of optional peppermint oil (you can make natural chocolate cupcakes if you wish).

½ teaspoon baking powder, sifted

¼ teaspoon sea salt

Chocolate mint curl glaze (contains dairy products)

one cup of butter at room temperature (2 sticks)

4 ounces of cream or chevre cheese (pour any liquid), room temperature; It's okay to replace GAPS with butter

⅓ Cup of sweetener of your choice: Confectioners for Keto

(or Stevia to taste), honey for GAPS, honey or maple syrup for Primal

3 tablespoons of Fairtrade cocoa powder, see recipe information

1 teaspoon of peppermint oil, see recipe notes; The intensity of the brands varies. So read the recipe notes for the brand or try the amount if using a different brand.

½ teaspoon spirulina (optional) see recipe instructions OR use beetroot powder or natural food coloring for pink icing

PREPARATION

Muffin

Preheat the oven to 325 degrees Fahrenheit. Place the tins in the muffin tins. Put aside.

Put the warm (not cold) liquid ingredients in a large bowl at room temperature and mix in the following: coconut butter (sweetener if you are making GAPS or a variation of maple syrup), melted coconut oil, eggs, whole milk, and optionally peppermint with mint oil.

also In a medium bowl, whisk the dry ingredients together: sweetener (if you're making the keto or coconut sugar version), cocoa powder, coconut flour, gelatin, baking powder, and sea salt.

Add the dry ingredients to the wet ingredients. Stir to combine; Don't mix too much. Pour about 2 ounces of batter into each muffin slot.

then start by Baking in the preheated oven for 25 minutes. Try baking with a toothpick. Look for moist, sticky crumbs. Take out of the oven. Fresh.

Chocolate and Mint Swirl Glaze

Put in a large bowl: butter at room temperature and cream cheese at room temperature. Use the mixer on high speed for beating well until the consistency is clear, about 30 seconds.

Add your favorite sweetener and keep whisking until everything is well incorporated.

Add the peppermint oil and the spirulina optioanl. Mix again until everything is completely incorporated. Gather half or a little less than half of the frosting in the center (be sure to set it aside) of a piping bag (or all of it in a piping bag if you want to put 2 full piping bags in a third piping bag to close the hot tub create)).

Add cocoa to the bowl with the icing. Beat to mix until completely incorporated. Fill the second half of the piping bag with chocolate icing. (or fill the second piping bag with chocolate icing).

Pour the frosting over the cooled cupcakes. Help!

25
KETO LEMON POPPY SEED MUFFINS – MOIST

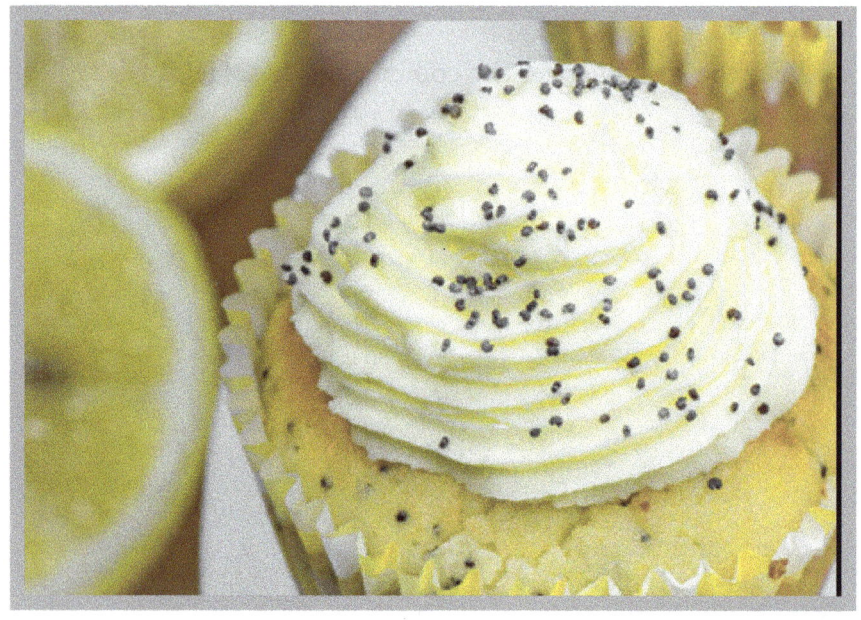

1 HOUR

Servings 12

INGREDIENTS

Magdalena

2 cups of almond flour

2 teaspoons baking powder

1/3 cup granulated, non-powdered normal erythritol

2 large eggs

1 cup sour cream

1 teaspoon vanilla extract

1 tablespoon of poppy seeds

1 lemon zest and juice

Nail polish

4 ounces unsalted butter

1 tablespoon of lemon juice

1/2 cup erythritol powder

2 tablespoons of cream

PREPARATION

Preheat the oven to 180 ° C.

Put all the muffin ingredients in the blender and blend over medium-high heat for 3 minutes until just combined.

Pour 12 hole batter into muffin pan lined with cupcake paper. Fill each sheet ¾ completely.

Cook for 20-25 minutes until a skewer comes out clean through the center.

Let the cupcakes cool on a wire rack.

While the cupcakes are cooling, add the butter and lemon juice to the blender.

Mix at low temperature by adding the Natvia glaze with the

spoon. Add the cream.

Stir on medium speed until ingredients are fluffy and pale.

Carefully pour mixture into a piping bag and pour over cooled cupcakes. Enjoy!

Observations

nutrition

Serving size: 100 g | Calories: 241 kcal | Carbohydrates: 5 g | Proteins: 6 g | Fat: 23 g | Saturated fat: 9 g | Cholesterol: 69 mg | Sodium: 32 mg | Potassium: 125 mg | Fiber: 2 g | Sugar: 2 g | Vitamin A: 443 IU | Vitamin C: 5 mg | Calcium: 111 mg | Iron: 1 mg

26

GRAIN FREE TOASTED COCONUT CUPCAKES

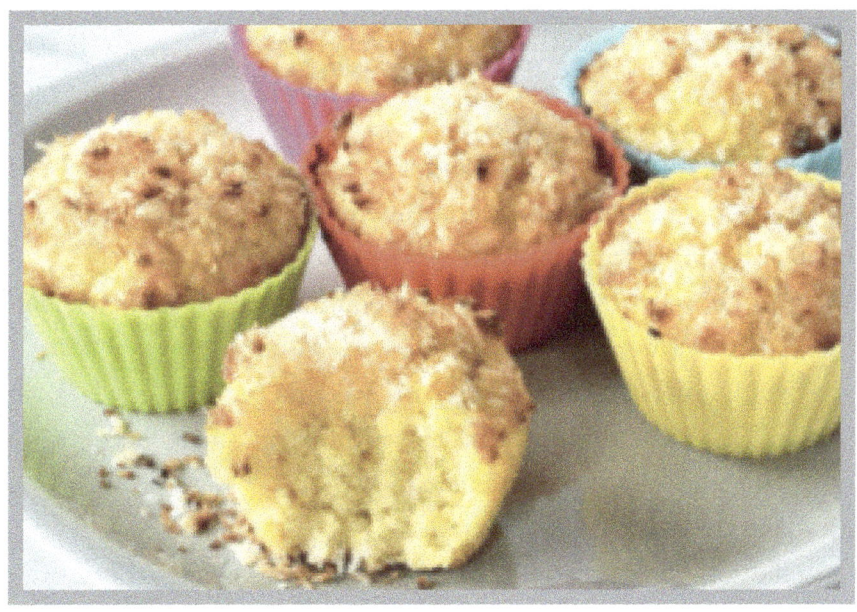

20 MINUTES

Servings 4

INGREDIENTS

Mass

1/4 cup butter, melted

3 eggs

3 tablespoons coconut sugar or your favorite sweetener

1 teaspoon vanilla extract

1/4 cup coconut flour

1/4 cup unsweetened dry coconut

1/4 teaspoon baking powder

1/4 teaspoon of salt

Coverage

1-2 tablespoons of unsweetened dried coconut to decorate

PREPARATION

Preheat the oven to 400 degrees.

start In a medium bowl, combine melted butter, eggs, sweetener, and vanilla with a whisk.

Add the coconut flour, dried coconut, baking powder, and salt to the wet ingredients and mix well.

Evenly fill six muffin cups or silicone muffin bowls with batter. Don't forget to grease the muffin tins if necessary. Top each cupcake with dried coconut.

Bake the cupcakes for 15 minutes.

take off cupcakes out of the oven and allow them cool completely before serving.

27
BROWNIE CUPCAKES WITH CREAM CHEESE FROSTING

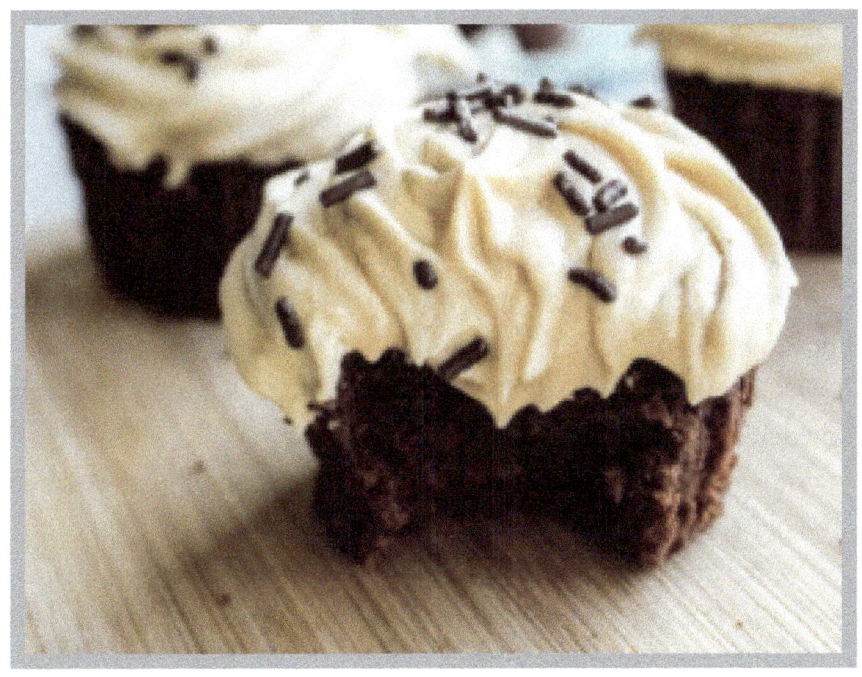

20 MINUTES

Servings 12

INGREDIENTS

1/2 cup almond flour
1/4 cup unsweetened cocoa powder
1 teaspoon of baking powder
1/4 teaspoon salt
4 ounces unsweetened chocolate, chopped
1/2 cup So nourished grainy erythritol
1 1/2 teaspoons vanilla extract divided
1/4 teaspoon of liquid stevia extract
5 large eggs
half package (8 ounces) cream cheese, softened
1/2 cup of this nourished erythritol powder
3/4 cup unsalted butter
3 tablespoons unsalted butter, softened

PREPARATION

Turn the oven to 325°F and prepare a muffin tray with paper liners.

In a mixing bowl, add almond flour, cocoa powder, baking powder, and salt.

In a small saucepan, combine ¾ cup butter and unsweetened chocolate.

When the chocolate and butter are melted, mix them gently, then add the granular erythritol, 1 teaspoon vanilla extract, and the liquid stevia extract.

take it from heat and let cool for 5 minutes.

After cooling, add the eggs one at a time, then add the dry ingredients until a homogeneous mixture is obtained.

Pour the batter into the prepared pan and fill it about 2/3 full.

Bake the cupcakes for 16-20 minutes until a knife inserted in the center comes out clean, then cool to room temperature.

To make the icing, cream together the cream cheese and the remaining butter.

Freeze the cupcakes as desired after gently whisking the erythritol powder and half a teaspoon of vanilla extract together.

28
KETO VANILLA BEAN CUPCAKES

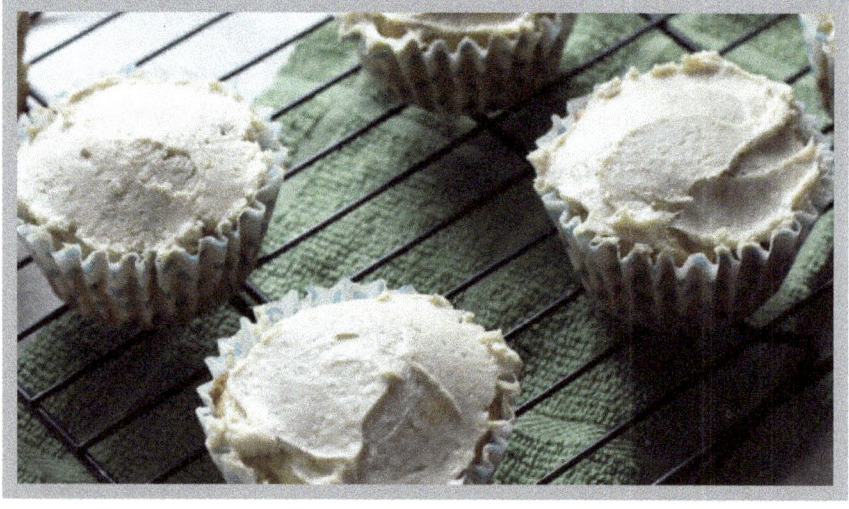

30 MINUTES
 Serving 4

. ..

INGREDIENTS

Cupcake Batter

2 large eggs

½ cup mayonnaise

1 tablespoon vanilla bean paste

1 ¾ cups almond flour

½ cup erythritol

¼ teaspoon salt

2 teaspoons baking powder

Vanilla Cream Cheese Frosting

4 ounces cream cheese

¼ cup powdered erythritol

3 tablespoons heavy whipping cream

½ teaspoon vanilla extract

PREPARATION

While collecting your ingredients, preheat the oven to 350° F.

Combine the eggs, mayonnaise, and vanilla bean paste in a medium mixing cup.

If necessary, use a hand mixer to make the batter completely smooth. Remove the bowl from the table.

Combine the almond flour, erythritol, salt, and baking powder in a separate dish.

Whisk the batter into the almond flour slowly. If you're having trouble putting them together, simply use a hand blender until they're smooth.

It's natural for the mixture to appear dry after it's been mixed.

Spoon eight servings into a lined muffin or cupcake pan using a 14 cup count.

Bake at 350°F for 20-25 minutes, or until lightly browned on top. After t, frost

KETO MAPLE CREAM CHEESE PUMPKIN MUFFINS

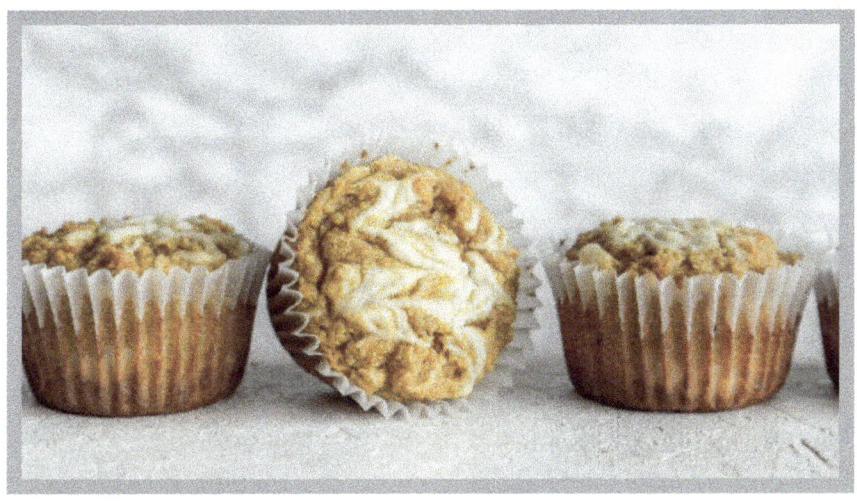

40 MINUTES
Servings 6

INGREDIENTS

Pumpkin Muffin:
1 cup almond flour, blanched
2 tablespoon coconut flour
1/4 cup stevia/erythritol blend
2 teaspoon ground allspice
1/2 teaspoon baking powder
1/4 teaspoon salt
2 large egg
4 tablespoon unsalted butter
2 tablespoon pumpkin puree
1/2 teaspoon liquid stevia

Maple Cream Cheese Filling:
2 ounce cream cheese, softened
1 teaspoon sour cream
1 teaspoon maple extract
1/4 teaspoon liquid stevia
2 teaspoon heavy cream

PREPARATION

All of the ingredients should be collected and packed. Preheat the oven to 350 degrees Fahrenheit.

Almond flour, coconut flour, stevia/erythritol mix, allspice, baking powder, and salt are all combined in a dish.

Combine the wet ingredients in a separate bowl: melted butter, eggs, pumpkin puree, and liquid stevia. Mix until it is well blended.

Combine the wet and dry ingredients in a mixing bowl and stir until smooth.

Whip the softened cream cheese in a separate bowl with a hand mixer.

Mix in the sour cream.

Pour in the heavy cream, maple extract, and liquid stevia. Mix all together until it's fully smooth.

Cupcake liners can be used to line a muffin tray. Half of the pumpkin muffin mixture should be included in each cupcake liner. On top of that, spoon the maple cream cheese mixture.

After that, add more pumpkin batter. Then, once again, top with the maple cream cheese mixture.

Mix these together with a toothpick to make a swirl. After that, bake for 25-30 minutes in the oven.

When the muffin is finished, a toothpick inserted into the center should come out clean. Take pleasure in it.

30
KETO NUTELLA: SUGAR-FREE HAZELNUT SPREAD

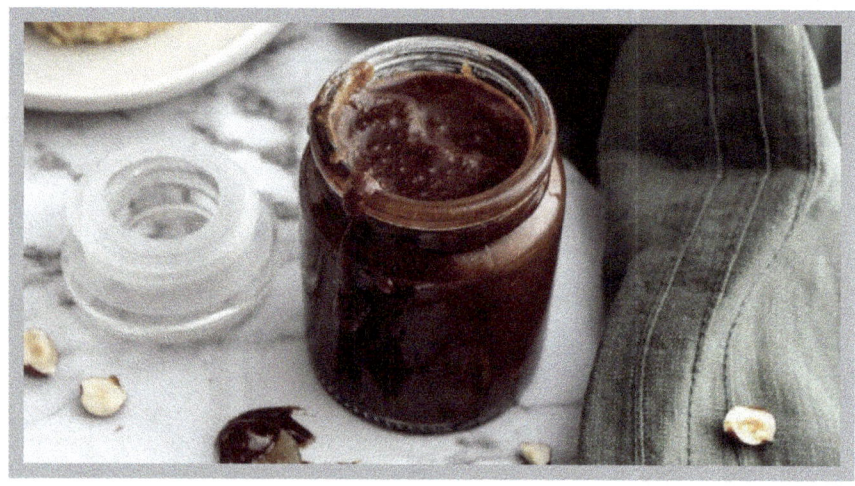

20 MINUTES
   Serving 32

INGREDIENTS

2 cup hazelnuts, raw

1/2 cup erythritol/stevia mix, powdered

1/4 cup cocoa powder

2 tbsp avocado oil

1 tsp vanilla extract

PREPARATION

Preheat the oven to 400 degrees Fahrenheit. Using parchment paper, line a baking sheet.

Hazelnuts should be spread out on a baking sheet. Roast for 8-10 minutes, or until golden brown and fragrant.

Place the hazelnuts in a resealable container with the lid on and shake vigorously once they have cooled slightly.

Repeat the procedure until all or almost all of the hazelnut skins have been extracted. Alternatively, you should rub the skins off yourself.

In a food processor or blender, combine the hazelnuts. Process for 2-3 minutes, scraping down the sides as needed, until the nuts start to form a nut butter. Combine erythritol/stevia blend powder, cocoa powder, avocado oil, and vanilla extract in a mixing bowl. Process for another 1-2 minutes, or until the mixture resembles a smooth spread. The spread should be silky smooth.

Taste and change the sweetener as needed. You can add 2-3 drops of liquid stevia at a time before you reach the desired sweetness stage. Enjoy! Store in an airtight jar for up to a month.

www.ingramcontent.com/pod-product-compliance
Lightning Source LLC
Chambersburg PA
CBHW071117030426
42336CB00013BA/2127